# THE ACCIDENTAL INDIES

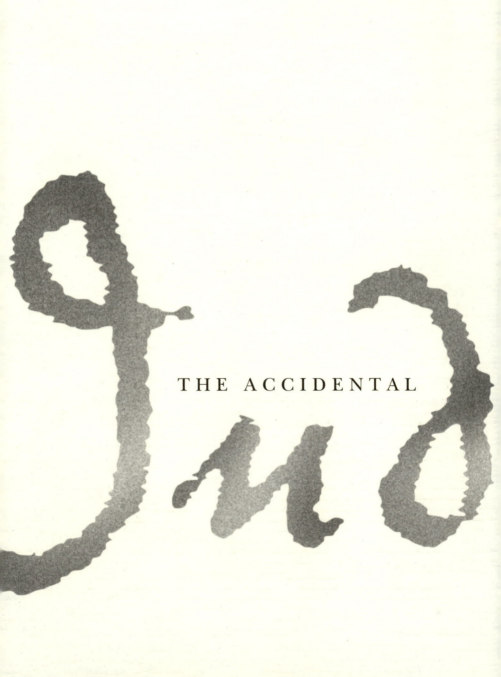

THE ACCIDENTAL

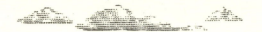

ROBERT FINLEY

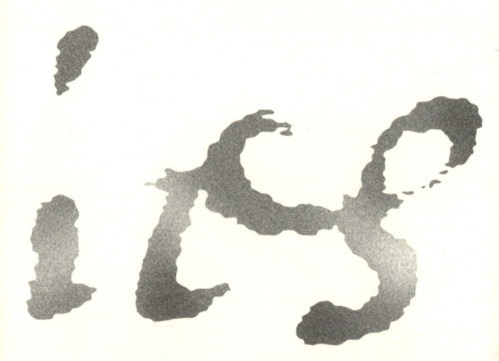

McGILL-QUEEN'S UNIVERSITY PRESS

Montreal & Kingston • London • Ithaca

© McGill-Queen's University Press 2000
ISBN 0-7735-2006-6

Legal deposit second quarter 2000
Bibliothèque nationale du Québec

Printed in Canada on acid-free paper

McGill-Queen's University Press acknowl-
edges the financial support of the Govern-
ment of Canada through the Book Publishing
Industry Development Program (BPIDP) for
its activities. We also acknowledge the support
of the Canada Council for the Arts for our
publishing program.


**Canadian Cataloguing in Publication Data**

.

Finley, Robert Stuart Martin, 1957-
    The Accidental Indies
    ISBN 0-7735-2006-6
    1. Columbus, Christopher–Fiction.
    I. Title.
    PS8561.15523A73 2000    C813'.54
    C99-901371-8
    PR9199.3f5314a73   2000


This book was typeset by Typo Litho
Composition Inc. in 10.5/16 Baskerville.

Designed by David Drummond

This book is dedicated to Ted Chamberlin

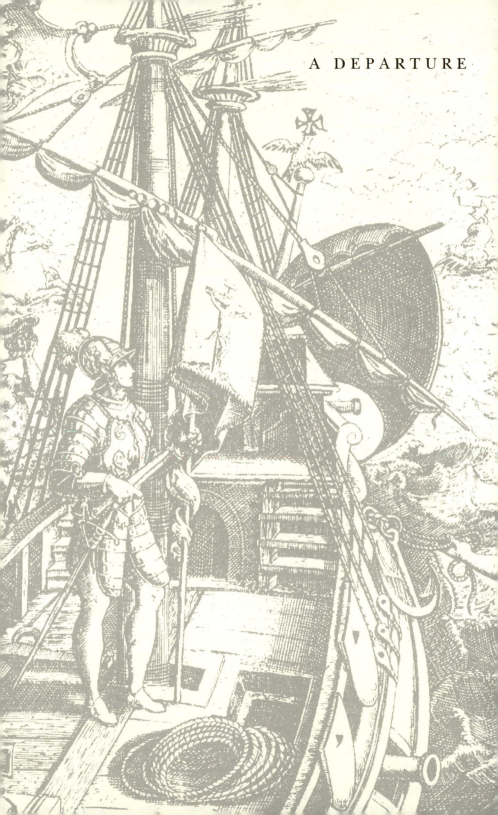

A DEPARTURE

... A hill there was, and on the hill a wide
extending plain, green with luxuriant
grass; but the place was devoid of shade.
When here the heaven-descended bard
sat down and smote his sounding lyre,
shade came to the place. There came the
Chaonian oak, the grove of the Heliades,
the oak with its deep foliage, the soft linden, the beech, the virgin laurel tree, the
brittle hazel, the ash, suitable for spear
shafts, the smooth silver-fir, the ilex tree
bending with acorns, the pleasant plane,
the many-coloured maple, river haunting
willows, the lotus, lover of pools, the ever-
green boxwood, the slender tamarisk, the
double-hued myrtle, the viburnum with its
dark-blue berries. You also, pliant footed
ivy, came, and along with you tendrilled
grapes, and the elm trees, draped with
vines; the mountain ash, the forest pines,
the abrate-tree, loaded with ruddy fruit,
the pliant palm, the prize of victory, the
bare trunked pine with broad leafy top,
pleasing to the mother of the gods, since
Attis, dear to Cybele, exchanged for this

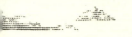

his human form and stiffened in its trunk.
Amidst this throng came the cone-shaped
cypress ...

So sang the nursemaid. And singing dreamt of
the place the song had made and of its cool green
shade. Her charge, however, had not been listening. Nor did he dream, but sat, his whole infantile
attention focused on her drooping eyelids, repeating over and over in his pre-articulate mind the
shape of "sleep, sleep ... sleep." And indeed,
whether by his wordless and insistent chant, or by
the mellifluous inflections of her own speech, she
slept and dreamt of the cool green shade the song
had made there, in the narrow room, in the summer heat of an afternoon in Genoa.

Hers is the first exit of our story. Even now the final moments of her employment as nursemaid and
guardian are racing by (racing, imagine, in the tor-
por of the afternoon). When she wakes everything
will be changed. Already the shadow of the foot-
steps that will in a moment thump up the stairs, the
final punctuation, the ellipses of her inattention, already the shadow of the first shoe is moving toward
the first step – though as yet she sleeps, content.
Hers is the first exit. Now, the first departure.

Her charge begins his earliest explorations, test-
ing the horizon of her sleep and his freedom in it.
While the nursemaid dreams, he's on the move.
Dimpled fists outstretched, he tries and worries the
obstacles of pillows, cases, blankets, his own unpre-
dictable infant self, the longitude and latitude of
his cradle, its desperate rocking – for, caught bril-
liant in the afternoon light that comes in at the
window and dapples the book in her hands, caught
in that light is the object of his enterprise. The
shiny gilt of, perhaps, a crucifix glints on the interior wall of that small room above the street in
which a woman sleeps in her chair, a book of poetry
in her hands, smiling, unaware, and in which a
child manages a chubby knee up over the precari-
ous wall of his confinement – his eyes fixed and
shining on the east.

Before anything happens, before the inevitable
happens, we should note here in the child the
sense not only of a destination but of a destiny, and
how the two are twisted in a single thread. He is
onto something big, it's true. Think of the terrible
energy of infants, and of how he may have lulled
the nursemaid (who really needs this job) to inattention and to sleep. There is a knowing air about
him, an aloofness, one leg, one arm, his head up

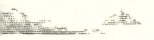

over the edge of his cradle. He, who has never been anywhere, seems already to be heady with that greatest of opiates, the here, here, here in there, the objective, journey's end. His mother named him for the burly pagan become saint, the ferry-man, Christ-bearer, simple man of a complex place, the carrier-across, Mr. Hither-and-Yon, the broad shoulders of the Word, Christopher: Χρο FERENS, Saint; and his father, no less caught up in the possible, gave him his other name, and the other half of fortune – Colon, arch coloniarch, or (from the Spanish) the dove of discord carrying in its beak a dead branch, a limb, a clause of itself across the wastes of seas, Colombo(us), bringer of news.

But we are being as inattentive as the poor nursemaid, whose two eyes, so recently shut and downward turning as twin crescents in a universal calm of sleep, are just now grown huge and dark, eclipsed by fright; she is pronouncing with them the startling letter "O!", come full awake to the telltale thud of ... but where is Christopher, and where has he been? We left him tottering on the unsteady edge of his infant world, bound, there's no denying, eastward. Since then our charge (the responsibility is at least partly our own) has, misjudging his distances, stepped out into the still and drowsy air of the afternoon and turned grace-

fully (if we slow him down, even artfully, even,
if we slow him right down, purposefully, even hero-
ically) turned four times head-over-heels before
coming up short against the rough boards of his
nursery floor. His course we can easily trace in the
whirling, gilded sun motes still spinning in the
gilded air. And so it is that Christopher first tested
the heft and roundness of this world against his infant head.

Let us retreat marginally from the scene to consider more carefully its geography. There is a westward window. Beside it sits a nursemaid, her face a
figure for astonishment and despair. Near her, a
large and somber cradle continues rocking omi-
nously and, like it a fleeting record of a recent ca-
tastrophe, a faint echo of this first and historic
conquest, the whorling sun motes begin to slow
and hang in the startled air. All else is still. The
room itself is bare, except, yes, to bless his name a
gilded crucifix hangs opposite the window, and at
this hour catches its light; from it a St Christopher
dangles on a chain. On the floor, between crib and
crucifix, lies the child. His eyes wide and tearless,
he is transfixed with – with what? – with a secret
pleasure? What he seeks is still beyond him, and he
holds it in a gaze so rapt that you, reader, might
concern yourself with his welfare; a concussion?

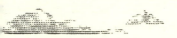

perhaps an imminent and swift ascent along the
bright trajectory of his upward gaze to his maker?
I'm here to tell you, he's all right. Columbus is
immune to distances.

All right?

The mother: "Oh my moon, my poor sweet
moon." She tends his poor bruised head.

The father: Intransigent.

It is only the nursemaid who understands that
the world has changed forever. (Harsh words have
been spoken; her prospects are bleak. Dismissed,
she is standing at the door of Uncertainties. She
feels sure it opens onto the street of Pain, so she
hesitates. But it's no good, and now – she's gone.)

And the world? The new names start to stir in
their shells. In (Virginia) a pigeon falls out of the
sky, which puzzles everybody who sees it. In the
(Yucatan) an unhusked cob of corn bursts into
flames for no reason. On (Hispaniola) a woman
gives birth to numberless snake children, and
on the islands north of there and south of there
and east of there and west of there everyone re-
members the origin of enemies. And in Europe,
the fortieth grandfather of the hemp seed that
will grow the first fibres twisted and knotted into
the log line of the Santa Maria is cut down with a
sharp scythe.

## WHO KNOWS WHAT TO EXPECT?

Bartholomew: Have you ever been to China?

Alonso: I don't know.

Here Christopher would surely say: "You don't know? Have you any reason to believe that you might have been there at some time?"

Alonso: (Silence)

Bartholomew: Were you, for example, ever near to the Chinese border, or were your parents there at the time when you were born?

Alonso: (Silence)

Christopher: Normally Europeans know whether they have been to China or not!

And so it is that, many years later, in their apartments in the city of Lisbon, Columbus and his brother Bartholomew mete out the thin soup of inquisitorial kindness, and with each spoonful the questions, the endless questions. Their house guest is not well. He is a sailor, Alonso Sanchez, and is at this moment as insubstantial as gossamer, nearly transparent with deprivation. To this can we credit the weakness of his responses, not quite audible over the centuries? The shadowy dinner guest has been brought home in a handcart from the docks where he appeared early this morning, gaunt and

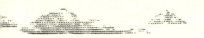

in rags. He claims that he is (for now) the sole sur-
vivor of an ill-fated voyage to England, that he was
blown westward, weeks westward from his course.
Columbus has had him put to bed by the fire,
where he has slept all day, his breathing weak and
uncertain, his secrets under his tongue. His hosts
pace anxious circuits round the room. Finally, curiosity outweighs charity and the soup is brought in
to the bedside, and with it the litany of questions:

Have you ever been to China?

The pilot is thinking about the apparition through
the fog of a steep headland. It is blue with spruce
wood, and sweet smelling. It is grace. Three weeks
before, he had felt the first warm twist in the swell-
ing gusts from the southeast, and all night the
ground swell building. And then the dreadful
chaos of morning on a sea changed utterly and in-
explicably out of itself. That wind lasted a week,
then came from the east. Four days later they
passed through its unsteady eye and fought their
way out of it for another week on the other side,
their ship flailing the broken seas like a drowning
man. Then, just at dusk, the wind dropped as
though it had no memory, and there it was, ghostly,
scented, just broaching the fog and looming beyond it, and the pounding of breakers. They stood

off for the night, holding that vision in the dreams of their exhausted sleep, and when morning broke, it was gone.

Alonso Sanchez dies in the night. Even the thin soup, after so long with nothing (drinking his own urine, sucking moisture from the entrails of certain sea-birds) was too rich. In the morning Columbus finds him, his eyes open but opaque, flat, no longer glittering with those vast distances. He closes them gently with his thumb and forefinger, and he sees that headland. But not only it. He traces the white line of the breakers with a thick pen, enclosing and naming the space behind it. This line he extends, tentatively, with a finer pen; to the south a rain of islands, to the north a long low shore. Cathay. There is great beauty in it, this abstract, its innocence, framing nothing but the essential shapes, leaving the rest. The questions were unnecessary. Columbus knows what to expect.

## WEST IS EVERYWHERE

Columbus knows what to expect because a letter is coming to him in the mail. It is coming by ship and takes a long time. He is impatient. He barely speaks to his young wife as they eat their dinner of rabbit

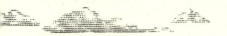

stew in the cramped house in desolate Porto Santo.
But here is the letter now, approaching by the
shore road. In a moment it will be in his hands. He
knows that it contains the best wishes of Paolo del
Pozzo Toscanelli, and also a map. The map will say,
"whatever you do you will meet with success." Columbus knows that he will succeed. The letter will
say "in so many leagues you can reach those places
most rich in all manner of spice, and of jewels, and
of precious stones." Columbus knows how many
leagues. And it will say "be not amazed if I call west
where the spice grows, for it is commonly said that
it grows in the east, yet who so steers west will always
find the said parts in the west, and who so goes
east overland will find the same parts in the east."
Columbus is not amazed. He is encouraged. He
has always known that the East was not a place but
a name for riches, and that the West was every-
where. Here is the letter now, brought by the blind
boy from the docks, breathless, his horse lathering.
Doña Felipa Perestrello y Moniz brings it to him.
He pushes aside the stew pot and bowls and spreads
it out on the table, and everything is just as he had
known it would be, even the City of Heaven with
its bridges of marble, and the golden roofs of
Japan.

But just how wide is the Ocean? How would you put it? Could you manage it in a small boat? How big around is the earth? You've seen it in miniature a thousand times: borne on a giant's shoulders, cracked in cartoons like an egg, cratered, batted, booted, ballooned. It's an old familiar, is the earth. And photographed – kite on the end of a heart string, oh blue blue gem of unspeakable beauty, home, belovèd, bright casement in an endless night. And flown over it, in parts. The Ocean, the Atlantic Ocean: six hours going west, seven going east. But I was hoping for a more tangible answer. How many inches is the earth? How many feet, heel to toe? How many yards, nose to finger tip, how many fathoms, head to sole, is a sea crossing? Does that count the up and down of the tides? Should we somehow include in our measure the endless sweep of the currents?

Even as it stands, it's not an easy question. Now, forget about a continent. And again, how wide is the Ocean Sea?

> *According to the philosophers and*
> *Pliny, the ocean which stretches be-*

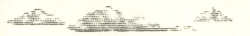

*tween the extremity of further Spain*
*and India is of no great width.*

Well that's good news. And Columbus, standing at
the reading table by the window in the house in
Madeira, marks the margin of *Imago Mundi* with the
sign of a

pointing hand, 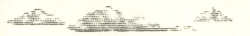, and reads on:

*An arm of the sea extends between*
*India and Spain.*
*India is near Spain.*
*The beginnings of the Orient and of*
*the Occident are close.*
*Water runs from pole to pole between*
*the end of Spain and the beginning of*
*India.*
*Aristotle [says] between the end of*
*Spain and the beginning of India is a*
*small sea navigable in a few days,*
*whence it follows that the sea is not so*
*great that it can cover three quarters of*
*the globe as certain people figure it.*
*The length of the habitable Earth on*
*the side of the Orient is more than half*
*the circuit of the globe.*

*Esdras says: "Upon the third day thou*
*dids't command that the waters should*
*be gathered in the seventh part of the*
*earth: six parts hast thou dried up,*
*and kept them, to the intent that of*
*these some being planted of God and*
*tilled might serve thee."*
*Observe the blessed Ambrose and Aus-*
*tin and many others considered Esdras*
*as a prophet.*

Why is he marking all these passages? Columbus
thinks that he is remembering something. In
fact, he is dismembering himself into marginal
notes. Even in his dreams everything is labelled
with the pointing hand: a horse running, ergo
the Idea; a house on fire, ergo the Idea; even
himself,

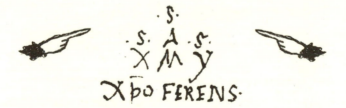

He is lost to it. Just look at him. Already it has
turned his hair white.

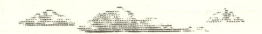

But let us follow the pointing hand further on. Where does it lead? Not just to these technical details of the ocean's brevity or the Orient's vast extent, bringing all the wealth of the East, so to speak, within its grasp. No, the pointing hand is more pervasive and more ambiguous than that. It leads us through a whole new world of marginalia: of fantasies, of grotesques, of titillations and taboos. Under its sign gathers the entire eccentric company of individual proofs that Columbus is now nurturing. This is not to say that membership in the Society of the Pointing Hand is not exclusive. Its requirements for sponsorship are as exacting as they are obscure. Whom else do we find here, courtly, gathered on the promenade? Who are these suave hidalgos of the margins who strut and turn in step to the guittern player and his muse? It is a very strange group indeed. Ocean Narrow and Orient Extent we have already met. Their dress is distinctly biblical, and their manner pontificating. They are always going on about the same thing, and often in chorus. Mostly they are avoided at all cost, except when a game is on – both terrible at cards, they tend to bet heavily. The big winner is usually El Dorado, gleaming, elegant, freshly powdered with gold, who, with his unlimited resources, keeps playing until he wins. Then there are the Cannibals.

"Naked as their mothers bore them," they come in from the margins of Marco Polo and Sir John Mandeville's *Adventures*, from Pliny's *Natural History*, the *Imago Mundi* of Pierre d'Ailly, and many others. Their habits are, of course, disgusting; not a dinner will pass under the sign of the Pointing Hand without one or another of them asserting wistfully that human flesh surpasses every other in the excellence of its flavour. But they are by far the largest group within this odd company of fellows, and they are the most engaging of the lot. One can always expect a warm welcome from the Cannibals. The Amazons (from the Island of Women), and the Men without Women (pale and severe from the Island of Men) keep pretty much to themselves, practising their swordplay on the east and west pistes respectively. From Polo too come the Men Born with Tails. Oh yes, and their relatives, from Angaman. Unspeakable, brutish, savage race of idolaters, they have the heads, eyes, and teeth of the canine species.

Before you, reader, scoff at the credulousness of our white-haired student of geography, bent at his table, now a candle burning beside him, his pen working in the margins of his books, or at this, his society of fellows, his marginalia, his beliefs, remember, all of these things were true. And you,

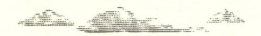

and I too, grew up in fear of the dreadful Anthro-
pophagi.

But what is the pointing hand that it can first
bring the land across the sea so near, and then populate it not just with riches but with this strange
company of grotesques? The pointing hand is no
less a thing than the constellation under which
Columbus will greet the unknown Other on the
shores of the New World; its brightest star is the star
called Wishful Thinking, and under its influence
we find that which we desire, the world as we desire
it. It is significant that it is not a hand armed, or a
fist clenched, or an open hand of greeting; it is the
pointing hand, the index, the finger that names,
decrees, instructs, and governs, the hand whose will
is fulfilled. The hand that points is magical: it has
the powers of levitation, of transformation, of cre-
ation and self-creation, and alas, of assimilation
and of extermination. It is not the loved one or the
friend that is pointed out with the pointing hand, it
is the thief in our midst, the pariah, the stranger.
The pointing hand is the final gesture of judicial
murder, of assassination, of genocide; it says,
"I name, I sentence." It is the great despoiler.

It is night. Columbus is working at his books. He
is fascinated by their subtle logic, how, under his
gaze, they seem to populate the empty reaches of

the heart with possibility and calm its solitary yearning. Then a noise in the street like the rustling of leaves distracts him, and I see that I have gone on too long. He moves from his desk, but it is a desk in Santa Fe and already it is 1492. At the window the stars are drifting westward and Spain is under the surgeon's knife, being bled. The Jews, carrying what they can, are streaming through the streets to the ancient ships, already crowded, of their exile.

Let us follow them to the sea.

## COLUMBUS' DREAM OF THE JOURNEY AHEAD

Columbus is in Palos de la Frontera, at the end of the road from Seville. The ships are nearly ready.

"And then I climbed up into the bows and called on the patron of all travellers to bless this undertaking, and on the heavenly name of our Lord Jesus Christ that he might, for the furtherance of Your Majesties and Your blessed enterprise, stand by me and aid me in its realization. And there one of the ship's boys was mending a frayed rope's end, and I had him climb up on the bulwarks and look out of the ship and tell me what he saw there. And he said, 'I see the river Tinto, sir, flowing softly to the sea.' 'And beyond that?' I said, and he answered, 'The

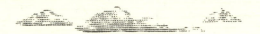

marsh grasses rippling, and the hill of Saltès, sir, and beyond, the Cross at Umbria.' 'And beyond that?' I said, and he answered, anxiously, 'The wastes of seas, as far as I can see, the Western Ocean like a whitening plain under heaven.' I called him down to me then and said, 'No, not the wastes of seas, but an infinite field for conquest. Look! You see there beyond the ocean stream a chain of islands to the south, and north a low extending shore, and a head-land steep with spice wood and sweet smelling, and there is a hill and beyond the hill a wide extending plain, and on the plain the mighty Tree on which our Lord was slain. The Indies, at the end of the western sea.'

"I could see then that I had calmed him, and I let him go about his work and myself went down again to my cabin. The afternoon sun slanted in at the porthole and lay across my hands and in my hands the book that I begin today, a record I thought to write all this journey in very carefully, from day to day, all that I might see and experience. The cabin was hot and drowsy, and while I was working these thoughts came to me, as though a dream. Everything was as it is, but changed. I was leaving a place to find out another, which tomorrow I will do. During the whole time of my travels, my eyes are shut, as they will be by mists and by the horizon of the heavy-lidded sea. When finally I arrive at my destination, the vision that greets me is, strangely, of this place, Palos. It is evening or morning, and the houses are aflame with the setting or the rising sun. A crowd is gathered on the dock waving in greeting or farewell, I cannot say, for instantly the vision flees, as though a candle had guttered and gone out. Then the sea is empty, and the horizon is again unbroken. Also it seems that my ship has turned to stone. I find I am weeping, and that the blood that streams from the deck of the stone boat into the endless sea is my tears. These thoughts were like a circle, though the journey was straight, and in my heart I felt the O of emptiness gathering as though the land I travelled in was a land of absences and I was left with nothing. For this I am afraid to sleep; until each day takes shape this emptiness consumes me. Now, facing west from this Spanish shore, I wonder what I started for so long ago."

## THE LABYRINTH OF DESIRE

The river is still greasy with night, and slow. It is half an hour before sunrise. Pale in first light, the moon at its quarter climbs down the western sky. The mooring lines slip heavily from the bows and

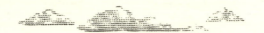

after a moment the current takes us. The river banks are wet with dew and the marshes brightening in the grey dawn. On the way out a fisherman hails us. We ghost by him, close enough to speak low, but there is nothing anyone can say or think of. In our dumb wake he throws the fine net with its margin of stones. It flashes a dark circle against the water. Then the ship's boy sings.

*Bendita sea la luz*
*Y la Santo Veracruz*
*Y el Señor de la Verdad*
*Y la Santo Trinidad*
*bendita sea el alma*
*Y el Señor que nos la munda;*
*bendito sea el dia*
*Y el Señor que nos lo envia*

By eight o'clock we take the tide up over the bar of Saltès and head out.

And you can see them now. Against a strong seabreeze they make their way forward, new rigging is tightened and retightened, the hills sink behind them. They stop at the Canaries and set out again, this time for the horizon only. But say, just say that the sceptics had been right all along, and that before them there was no real, no elemental sea, but only, after two, maybe three day's sail due west, the threshold of their understanding. Beyond it, despite the familiar passage of the days and nights, and the flight of the stars, say they venture into the Sea of Allegory. Before them the moon at its quarter swings down the western sky, and its chaste goddess of the hunt, Roman Diana, with her bow and quiver of plagues, walks at the ship's side, its bridle in her hand. Neptune with his trident and trinity of horses rides a Botticelli shell off to port, and scouts ahead. It is, after all, new territory for him as well. In the distance, are those islands, or clouds drifting up over the horizon into a false perspective? Sea sightings are often tricks of light, so close to the huge distorting lens of the bellied ocean. Except, yes, there they are again, just visible in the coat of arms that billows from the masthead. Sinister: anchors and a lion rampant; Dexter: a castle and the islands in the sea. That the ship is armed and cannon ready is no surprise, the sea pregnant with those shapes sea-monstrous, and there on deck is the coiled rope for binding and for bringing back. Close in to port, two lusty sea-centaurs blow a fanfare on their conch shells, while a pair of sirens off to starboard are promising a song. Columbus himself stands in the ship's centre, fully armed, out-

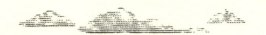

sized, one hand at his sword, in the other a staff
and Christian banner. He looks westward. Is it those
islands that hold his gaze, or the sirens singing, or
the standard of the Cross obscuring all? He seems
aloof. Does he, coursing into history, so disdain the
graceful progeny of his mythic heritage to leave
them in his wake? We've seen him in this state before, the fixed assertive look, the surety. And what is
that – out in front? Unsteady on the bowsprit the
eager dove, wings outstretched, articulates the
wooden letter of the Cross and prepares to fly.

What you cannot see in this picture are the huge
circling currents, the respiration of the whale, or
the whale's way turning and turning on itself, the
great ease of oceans around continents. The feathered coral feels it, the sand banks sketch it, the
seethe and drag of the tides knows it, but you cannot see it here. Nor can you see the round earth
made strange by the helmsman's good work, by the
charged hull, the lodestone, the Genoese needles
balanced on their axes, by the fine straight line
(the course is true) growing westward, dividing,
never turning back on itself, always moving westward.

Nor will you find here any of the icons of explo-
ration, no instruments of observation or of record.
The ship is ill-equipped, the islands are misty and

remote. He is naked in that armour, the Discoverer. Where does he think he is going?

WEST

The way west is the way east. The way out is the way in. At five, maybe six miles per hour the knotted thread is unwound to the centre of the labyrinth of desire. The heart is eager, it is violent, it is empty. The winds have turned and carry him effortlessly forward.

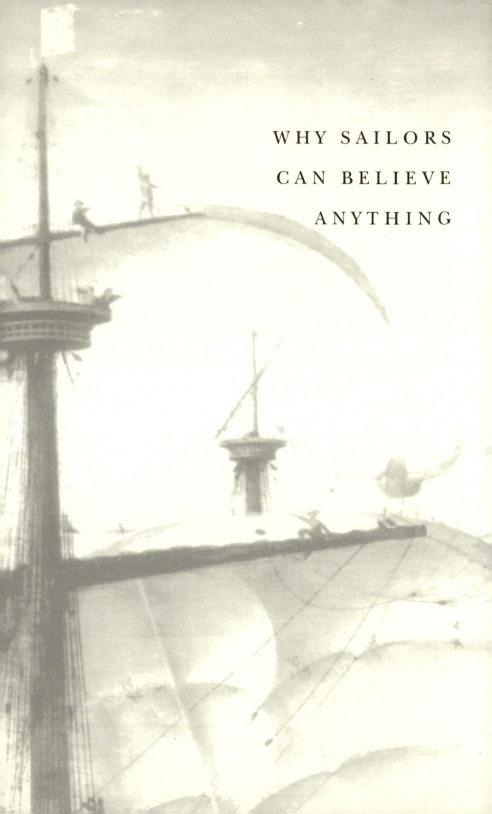

WHY SAILORS

CAN BELIEVE

ANYTHING

*andando más, más se sabe*
CHRISTOPHER COLUMBUS


If you had climbed the hill up behind the town, you
would have seen them there, three ships loitering
on the horizon, their sails slack, slatting half-heart-
edly with the ground swell. And if the next morning, Sunday morning, you had been on an errand
and passed by that hill path again, you might have
stopped for a moment to catch your breath – your
burden, some wool you have spun for the weaver in
the next valley, is heavy, and you put it down to rest.
And when you look up from the broken path and
out to sea, you say, "Ah, so now they have gone."
But where have they gone? No more than they
themselves can you imagine it. The helmsmen have
steered badly, the set of the currents is unknown,
and the logic of the stars and of the compass rose
there blooming under the navigator's gaze remains
obscure. With every day that passes, less and less
can be said of where they are, further and further
from the one fixed point, the mountain soil beneath your feet where you are stooping now to take
up your load and go on your way.

When the wind comes, it comes from the northeast and at night. It is brisk but sweet, and makes

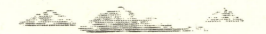

the heart beat both ways; it comes from home and
carries in its arms the shapes of the familiar, even
while the wake builds under the bows and broadens
astern. Departures are always the same. There is
the one wave that is the first and the last wave that
you notice, the first gentle lift and fall of the dark
hull under your feet. And with it the world falls
away from you quite suddenly and softly, like a
word you have spoken. Whatever your reasons for
setting out, a lightness and a loneliness gather under your heart. From now on the only rhythms are
the sea's rhythms and the only voice is the senseless
incantation of the waves. All about you gather the
distances; the remoteness of the stars is there only
to remind you of the unsoundable depths touched
by the narrow keel, and every morning opens
around you the perpetual horizon. After a few days
you start to forget. You forget what it was that
brought you out here, you forget to ask yourself
where you are, you forget where you are going. The
ship carries with it its own sense: the changing of
watches; working the pumps and sails; meals
around the daily hearth kindled at the ship's centre, backs against the bulwarks or rigging; talk. But
all of it, every movement, every gesture, is measured against the rhythm of the waves, which you

also forget so perfectly that finally they enter your dreams and you start to dream the same dream over and over and over.

The bright waters babble at the bows and out of the wind the sun is hot and drowsy. There is the gentle crushing of the waves and the spars' rhythmic creaking, and somewhere overhead a pennant drums irregularly against the taut cotton of the sails. The crew is busy at the windward rail; two grapnel lines snake out from the ship's side and their hooks dig deep into the flanks of a huge spar lolling half underwater, bearded with weeds. The sailors secure it, and as the ship rolls to leeward, the lines draw bar tight. On the second roll, the great tree itself lumbers sideways and shakes out the grappling irons. Then it is out of reach astern. Its head heaves out of the wave-wrack once and sinks back. A long way back in the ship's wake, you can see the waves, charged by its presence, breaking over it.

The old Majorcan waits until dark to begin: *Aixo era y no era* ... but everybody already knows that a huge sea snake came and fought with them; that finally it shook out the painful grappling hooks and slipped away astern; that it struck the rudder such a blow with its tail that the helmsman was thrown to

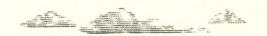

the deck – and look, has the bruises to show for it.
And that then it raised its bearded head once or
twice, and made the sea foam, and disappeared.
They know it was and was not so, because they
know that at sea things are always what they seem.
This is why sailors can believe anything.

The next morning the sailors find that they are
restless and watchful. All night they listened to the
rustling wake, and today they are waiting for something to happen. Everyone is waiting. Everyone is
watching the sea for signs. What do they find? They
find that the compass is not truthful; they find a
great fire that falls from the sky; they find dolphins;
they find dark clouds like islands to the north, and
to the south; they find the sea choked with weeds;
they find a whale; they find a contrary wind; they
find several times that they are mistaken when they
thought they had found land; they find birds, or
are found out by them – land birds, sea birds, song
birds, white birds, bright birds, birds with long tails,
birds that don't alight on the sea, birds that never
go far from land; they find a green reed, a carved
stick, and a branch with berries; and they find a
light that gutters and goes out.

Let us follow then, and from the vantage of our
own boat, that monument, the stone boat buoyant
in the current of time, from its decks and high win-

dows watch as they make their wandering way. We stand in now silently under their lee and take up with them their westward course. It is evening. The three ships scud along to windward, Columbus on his afterdeck.

〰

THURSDAY SEPTEMBER 13TH
*The compass does not point north.*

〰

His left hand rests on a low binnacle in front of him and follows the motion of the ship. His right, his arm outstretched, palm pressed flat against the northern sky, he holds steady, its own constellation fixed for a moment in the sphere of stars that gather faintly in the gathering dusk. His palm spans the dark lacuna of the night, and balanced exactly at the tip of his index finger, glimmering more and more brightly, is Polaris, the Pole Star, the fixed North, the True. But when he lowers his hand slowly from the darkening sky to the compass face where it rests like a shadow on the glass, he feels an itch of panic stir in his fingers and cross, twining at the palm and wrist. The needle does not point north, but, with its charged and figured end, north-and-askance, into the periphery of north. The pro-

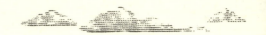

cedure is repeated. To take the north and mark it,
first find the North Star. Hold the right arm
straight before you, the palm of the hand facing
outward. Bring the star to the tip of the index finger, and then lower the hand steadily to the compass face, the axis of the needle nesting in against
the first knuckle of the first finger. Again the compass does not point True, and this time Columbus
feels the needle's lean balance, south, pointing ob-
liquely back not quite at, but toward him standing
there in his tiny ship, on a strange sea, as the night
comes down around him dressed in its rare mantle
of the most distant stars.

A ship at sea has one anchor to the world, its
direction. Snubbed into the last headland at its
point of departure, its course uncoils and
straightens along the lines we plot from port to
port. This time the compass varies only a few de-
grees, but this gap breaks the circle of the sailors'
trust in the laws that brought them out here and
were meant to take them back. Now, every inch of
ocean that passes under the thin planks carries
them further into a world that makes no sense.
Suddenly the night is full of voices, and they feel
the shadow touching them of an invisible presence that leaves messages they cannot read in-
scribed in the lodestone. Tonight everyone

dreams the same dream. In it everything is just as it is around us, the same sea, the same sky, the same ships, two together and one to starboard and a distance ahead. Everything is the same, even the sound of the pennant that thrums the topsail, everything, except when the day in their dream dawns, there is no horizon.

~~~

FRIDAY SEPTEMBER 14TH
*They see terns and a tropic bird, and these birds,*
*they say, never go far from land.*

~~~

When we wake it is to a new sea of emptiness, except for the birds. They fly along between the three ships and our own, a tropic bird rowing the wind at the mastheads, white, with a long reed tail, and some black hooded terns going west. Look at those terns, the orange of their beaks threading the blue waves. But already they are a sign for something else, transparent emissaries for an unnamed country just a day's run out of reach. Of course this is a mistake: it is the men, not the birds, that have never gone so far.

~~~

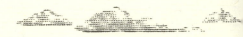

*A marvelous branch of fire falls from the sky into the sea
not far from the ships.*

And so they wait, poised like awkward birds in the
rigging, in the bows, at the sterncastle and helm,
until the next sign comes. We are standing at the
starboard rail of the stone boat, you and I, watching
the three ships off to windward trailing their white
wakes behind them under the dome of the night
sky, the dark shapes of their sails, the dark hulls cut
out of its starred cloth. Though tonight they are
making good time with all bonnets laced and the
spritsails flown, the following sea is easy, and the
night seems still. You turn in against the rigging to
light a cigarette, and then turn back and lean out
against the rail beside me, into the warm wind. We
are expecting it, of course, but still, just then, when
the three ships light up like that, like a premoni-
tion, it takes us by surprise. All the tracery of their
rigging and gear, the black hulls, the shadowy sails
awash with golden light, they seem to toss wildly
and burn, and the shadow of our own ship's spars
and towers is cast down across the burnished sea
before us. We turn with the rest and see in the
south-west the great branch of flame falling to the
sea not too far off.

On the three ships they all agree that it is a good sign, this ship of fire with its slow wake that arches over them (and over us in our ship of smoke and ashes) and hangs there for a moment from the domed ceiling.

"Strange, that no one seems afraid," you say, looking back across the water at their faces still turned to the fading light.

But within the closed circle of our sight, a world vaulted now by fire as well as darkness, the gentleness has not gone out of the night. The branch of flame is more astonishing than I had imagined, too. But in this silence we are neighboured to it and to the still living stars and the dark waters that embrace them.

You leave me there, old man, at the rail, staring off into the deeper darkness that the wind is bringing, the traces of tomorrow's rain clouds lengthening above us and above the tiny ships, each now like a distant point of light, ourselves somehow among them.

∿

MONDAY SEPTEMBER 17TH
*They see dolphins.*

∿

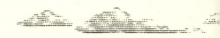

We see them first from far off. In a few minutes they cross the path of the three ships and turn from their way to play under the bows, and to lead them. By day as quick as shadows, by night they mine the living veins of light under the bow waves and ignite the dark water deep below the hulls. Dolphins: Delphinus delphis, the womb-fish, their constellation speeds westward with Pegasus, the Eagle, and the Arrow in its starred wake.

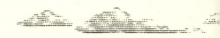

TUESDAY SEPTEMBER 18TH
*A large mass of cloud appears in the north,*
*which is a sign of being near land.*

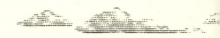

And to the south too there are the ghosts of islands we are sailing through – to starboard, black-backed Antilla, the Island of the Seven Cities: Aray, Ary, Vra, Jaysos, Marnlio, Ansuly, Cyodne; and to port the Fortunate Islands of Saint Brendan: the islands of Crows, of Rabbits, of Doves, the island of the Goats, The Wolf, San Zorzo, Ventura, and Brazil.

Just listen to them – the Ante Yllas, the Island that is Nowhere but Elsewhere; and in the other direction the blessed islands of the gentle Saint

Brendan, each one familiar, each a blessing of the earth. The sailors imagine rolling hills broaching the sea-wrack all around them, woodlands, fields of flowers, the scented wildrose and shapely lark-spur. On these smooth shores they let their hopes climb up, and they make their thanksgiving there. In their hearts the festive fire is already burning in the hearth. But, as though under the burden of their desires, the imagined islands sink and slip away, and the horizon opens around them once again. Columbus will turn neither to the north nor to the south, but keeps to his westward course.

Does he doubt the islands' presence there, just a few leagues off? Not at all. Even now they are touched, in his mind, by the broadening wake of the three ships. He has been expecting them all along. They are on the chart and on Behaim's globe, and what Behaim and the cartographers propose, Columbus knows. This is his great strength: he is a literalist of the imagination.

Columbus' chart is simple, but chart reading is a wary art. Even maps of the familiar are not easy to interpret. Things do not appear in their own shapes: they are translated into a code of skeletal elevations and outlines, elaborated with arcane

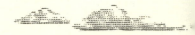

symbols – and they are pictured from above. What the navigator sees, both in the chart and all about him, is a cautious distortion. He anxiously bends his sight from the looming shadow of land – headland, island, cliff or beach – and turns the chart to meet it. Good navigators are always skeptical, not of the presences of things, but of what they see and understand. Good navigators are always almost lost. But Columbus is a visionary, and visionaries are not good navigators. The world they inhabit is the much simpler world of what they simply know. So the ships carry on unaware of the absences that brush by them on either side. The islands are not there, though the clouds attest to them. All of it, except the sea itself and the sailors' yearning, is an illusion.

〰

### THURSDAY SEPTEMBER 20TH
*Two or three land birds come to the ship singing.*

〰

### FRIDAY SEPTEMBER 21ST
*At dawn they find so much weed that the sea appears to be solid with it. They see a whale.*

〰

At first the sailors are delighted: the day is thick with possibilities. Everything points to "Land is Near."

But the sea bears looking at. Here they first find hope, and then, like a shining palimpsest, beneath their hope they read despair. They swing the lead and at two-hundred fathoms – all the line they have – no bottom. (Nor would the dipsey touch bottom at 2,000.) The realization creeps into them through the soles of their feet, like cold. It snakes up behind the eyes and looks out, and now the matted weed seems to hold them back.

Perhaps it is a sudden claustrophobia from the clinging weed, or morbid speculation on the whale that sets it off. Columbus staggers on the deck. Although he is standing in the clear bright air of afternoon, he feels confined and short of breath, as though he were entombed within the dank hold of the rolling ship. His vision blurs, his tongue is thick and heavy. Around him he feels presences that press against him, black shapes that crouch, or lie, or sit; they lean and cling, half effaced within a dim and sallow light. He falls against the rigging. After a moment the dizziness passes, and when he looks up the water is still glassy and dilated where the whale has broken through the dull sargasso and sounded.

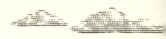

All that night the sailors, and we with them, watch the St. Elmo's fires catch up and pass by to leeward burdened with their black cargo, the night. And sleeping close by the hull, they hear the weeds whisper along the ships' flanks. Some think that it is the distant singing of birds that they hear, others that it is the voices of their drowned fathers, still others think that the children of Atlantis are crying out to them as they pass over. The whales are calling, it is true. But not to them.

*SATURDAY SEPTEMBER 22ND*
*The wind blows from the west and against them*
*for the first time.*

Increasingly the sailors imagine that when they speak even their own shipmates cannot hear them, their words carried off and cast up months later on a foreign shore, broken by the east wind. Even when they dream of home, they move through its familiar streets and rooms unable to speak or cry out to those around them, their speech entangled by the awful distances they have been travelling in. Every morning is fine, perhaps a few clouds late in the day, perhaps a light rain,

and everyday there is that sweet steady breeze out
of the east that whispers fantastic distances into
the ships' logs; the squat big bellied hulls slide
down the steep sides of the following sea. But as
the weight of days masses up at their backs, they
discern something sharp and sour on the air. Just
faint at first, it teases at the threads of their anxi-
ety, already taut and shrill behind them. Then
they recognize it: it is the smell of a ship on the
homeward passage, its crew gaunt and staring, the
sails blown out, the decks opened in the heat, the
barrels sprung, the bilges foul after weary months
at sea, the wind still contrary.

Square-rigged ships go in only one direction:
they go downwind, irrevocably. So when the wind
does come, for a day or two, from the west with a
building sea, it slows their progress but speaks a
greater comfort than any of the signs of land.
"Such a thing had not been seen since the time of
the Jews, when Egypt came out against Moses who
was leading them out of captivity," writes Columbus
in his log. He is exaggerating, but he looks relieved.

Soon the pennants again point to the west, and
again the waves part at the bows and babble along
the ships' sides – and the promised course is again
made true.

∿

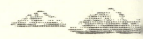

SUNDAY SEPTEMBER 23RD
*They see a dove, a booby, a small river bird,*
*and other white birds.*

ᗜᗜ

TUESDAY SEPTEMBER 25TH
*The captain of one of the caravels sees land.*
*The sailors on all three ships climb the masts and*
*into the rigging and all affirm that it is land …*

ᗜᗜ

But it isn't.

How simply desire invades and corrupts the navigator's art! Tomorrow afternoon the sailors will go swimming in it, this chimera, this trick of light and shadow, this land. They will dive from the high bulwarks and rigging, make graceful arching dives out from the ship's side, they will dive deep and surface white and unscathed on a sea smooth and forgetful as a river all around us. They will let their white limbs carry them out from the dark hulls onto the lift and fall of the ground swell and float there buoyed up by the invisible current, their arms outstretched, miles above the ocean floor.

Columbus retrieves his chart from the captain of the caravel and makes the necessary adjustments, not to it, but to the world he is sailing in. The sea allows this, it even invites it.

~~~

FRIDAY SEPTEMBER 28TH
*They catch two dorados.*

~~~

And you too, old man, have brought out your bag of hooks and line, and let the weighted jig sink into the shadow of the stone boat. Its shiny lure glints less and less distinctly as it travels down through the regions of the sea, one below the other. After you sit there for a while, jigging, the line thrills like a nerve all the way back to the synapse of your hand held over the water, and I can see that you are understanding something. Suddenly you are the root we are rooted to, the swaying ship, its rigging, myself, the unbearable distances which surround us, suddenly it is all fixed by the trilling wire leading down into the dark water. What is it you are fishing for, I wonder.

~~~

SATURDAY SEPTEMBER 29TH
*They see three boobies, and four tropic birds.*

~~~

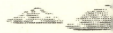

### MONDAY OCTOBER 1ST
*There are rain squalls.*

∿

The squalls begin in the morning; we watch them approach, lifting over the horizon's lip on their black wings. Slanting shafts of rain crowd in around us until the whole circle of our sight is like a pillared hall. The three ships appear and disappear all day among its shifting columns. Toward evening there is a break in the clouds which lets down shafts of light as well. We thread our course among them.

∿

### THURSDAY OCTOBER 4TH
*Forty petrels come to the ship all at once, and two boobies,*
*one of which the ship's boy hits with a stone. Also, a frigate bird*
*and a white bird like a gull come near.*

∿

### TUESDAY OCTOBER 9TH
*All night they hear the birds passing.*

∿

He rarely sleeps at night, Columbus. The night is too precipitous, opening over and over again onto shadow islands and ghost continents. Sometimes he dozes during the day, once the dependable O of the horizon has hardened around them in the morning light, and often he will lie down on his bunk for an hour in the evening to rest his eyes. He is there now.

All night, beyond the familiar creaking of the ship, the jabbering of the waves, and the officer's low murmured commands to the helmsman, they hear the birds passing. Flock after flock flies over them, moving south-west. In the darkness, their wings touch the sails and brush past the rigging. The lookout at the mast-head feels their weight as they lift over him, and below in his cabin Columbus hears them, constant as heartbeats. They lead him into sleep, and in his sleep he follows them. He dreams that he is coasting a wooded shore line. He has come upon it suddenly in a rain squall and can see maybe a mile of it laid out before him. He thinks he recognizes it from his chart; at the very least it breaks up into coves, bays, islands, or begins the long curve of a continent – the coast of Ciamba? of Moabar? But it is the Coast of Contradictions he is dreaming of. He starts south along its long low shore and loses the dark line of the trees in the dusk. He is carried off-shore in the cool and muscular currents of a huge

river in whose waters he detects an unearthly pu-
rity. All night he tacks into heavy weather, out and
back, out and back, until suddenly he comes up
short. Out of the darkness, a hundred yards off,
looms a steep headland. With dawn, he intuits a
connection between landfalls and traces it on his
chart of fragments. But he doubles back in day-
light – perhaps he has overlooked a blind bay behind the inscrutable line of palms that line the
beach, or a narrow channel that squints into a harbour the size of a world. Then he notices that
there are people among the trees, hundreds of
people, naked, standing perfectly straight and
still, their backs turned toward him, looking into
the blue-dim forest. They too are facing west. But
they are looking into it.

Columbus tries to see past them, and beyond
the curtain of the trees. He draws close in under
the shore and immediately the boat he is travelling in, which had been sound, and his compan-
ions, who had been singing in the shrill voices of
children, begin to change. The boat is full of
holes, and begins to sink, and the children who
had been singing are reduced to a dull percussion
of bones that clatter as they fall, bone against
bone, into the boat. Now he is alone. The ship set-
tles like a stone on the sandy bottom of a shallow

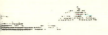

bay that lies within the crescent of a white beach he cannot reach or cross. Beyond the beach the feathered palm trees wave to him in greeting, or, with their feathered lances, in warning, he cannot say. People come out of the dark forest to give him things – they swim out with long, sure strokes to bring him food to eat, water in gourds to drink. Sometimes they come to the edge of the forest and yell with shrill cries and shoot at the ship with their bows. The tiny wooden arrows clatter harmlessly about him, against the masts and rigging. Sometimes they come and seem to beckon him and call to him to follow, to follow them into the wood. At first, at night, the stars spin crazily overhead, and all day he listens to the senseless lapping of the waves along the shore. Gradually, in his solitude, he thinks that he is making sense of them, of the stars, the currents, the white strand, and that he belongs there on that littoral. A voice on the other side of waking keeps saying, no, no, you are not making sense of them, you are lost. That is the sound of the birds flying over, their one and perpetual home under the span of their wings. They lead him toward waking, and at dawn, he alters his course to follow them.

~~~

*They complain of the long voyage. Then they see a green*
*bulrush near the ship, and take on board a carved stick,*
*and a piece of cane, and a small plank. They also see*
*a branch of roseberries.*

When morning comes and the horizon, unbroken,
still surrounds us, the sailors on the three ships can
bear it no longer. Each token they found along the
way seemed to point to land; now they suspect they
were signs for something else – the mast, bearded
by months, perhaps years at sea. But the stick has
been carved, it appears, with an iron knife, and the
branch is still green, and heavy with its red berries,
and the flocks trail westward.

*At ten o'clock at night, the Admiral sees a faint light*
*that is like a candle raised and lowered.*

This in the sensitive periphery of sight where even
the faintest glimmer will show itself. When we turn
toward it, it is gone. The light is the last sign, but
neither it, nor any of the other signs can be
charted, and even here in the last moments of the

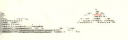

outward voyage we can only speak broadly about
the sea or our place upon it. But let us use the flick-
ering light for a moment to look forward. In a few
hours the chaste moon will rise behind us and illu-
minate a white cliff and low shore a distance ahead.
At the moment of the lookout's cry from the mast-
head, wing-backed Pegasus, with Deneb in the
Northern Cross brandished before him, will de-
scend the night's steep bank among the western
stars and touch the western horizon with one hoof.
And behind us in the east, Jupiter will be rising
amid his flights of birds.

Morning will find us at anchor within the mouth
of a broad and shining bay where along each shore
the palm trees rustle and sway. Thirty-three days
out from the island of Gomera, the three ships'
boats will notch the bright auricle of the beach,
and the sailors will take their first unsteady steps
across the blessed horizontal of the sand. They will
mark the place with a cross hewn from an island
pine, its squared trunk flowering the scented flowers, their bone-white petals, cut by the steel
tongued adze. (Already in their sleep the carpenters rehearse the catechism of square and plumb.
Here, soothed by the perfumed air, the solace of
the flowers and the earth, and the clear water tast-
ing neither of vinegar nor the casks, they will speak

in voices that, after the roar and babble of a month at sea, seem strange to them, as though from long disuse. Here, standing in the tree's crossed shadow, they will pronounce the new name for the place, and although at first their voices are lost in the crush crush of the waves along the beach and echo strangely from the chambered woods behind it, singing, they will mark it in the air. Just like that will the dreamed-of place be known.

That is tomorrow. Tonight we are still at sea and even now, somewhere in the darkness out before us the beach is asking its eternal question. It is the same question that it asks and asks of all the waves that lisp along it – listen, listen. The sailors do not hear it yet. They do not hear it yet.

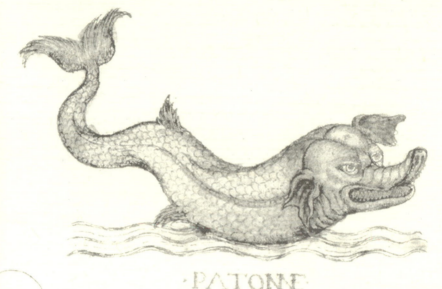

·PATONE·

Est ung poisson fort Excellent a menger
Aiant legoust dun esturgien et habitent
souvent aux riuieres doulces ;

THE ACCIDENTAL INDIES

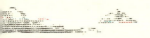

Already at first light, Columbus is at his table in the
gallery under the aft deck. The burnished vellum is
spread out before him, pinned flat, and all around
him arrayed in trays and cases are his pens and
inks, raw pigments, sable brushes, bottles of fine ab-
sorbent sand, his mortar and pestle, dividers in a
leather sheath, his rules and compasses. Yesterday
he prepared a ground of gum arabic to coat the
hide and let it dry in the east wind that swelled all
afternoon behind them. Now, as they make their
way in, the ship steadying when it finds the line of
the island's shelter and the ground swell suddenly
subsides, he leans against the table and inscribes a
figure for the journey itself, a kind of invocation,
the compass rose.

It is clear that he has laboured over the stencil.
Here, at the centre, are the petals of a flower in
perpetual bloom, this circled by a band of gold
leaf on which are set eight indigo diamonds, one
for each of the world's eight winds. Around these
runs a horizon of plain black bordered by threads
of cochineal. And from the rose's centre he has
drawn out thirty-two fine straight lines, black por-
tolan lines, that emanate across the whole plain of
the vellum like the rays of a darkened sun, a cloud
drawn across its face. This process he repeats
around the chart's perimeter, each rose oriented

to the others, their rays criss-crossing to form a loose net, weighted at the edges, for his observations. And here, leaning in from the margins, the faces of four wind gods animate the empty space between them, their cheeks straining, their hair caught back in invisible gusts.

Why are charts so wonderfully engaging? He works in a sort of rapture, does Columbus, despite the busy ship around him, now pauses to trim his pen, and now stoops again to the table, narrowing his gaze. And I must confess, I too have felt their beauty, their allure, and spent my share of hours bent over a broken-backed atlas tracing with my finger the road or river furthest north or south or east or west, or indeed, a mazy course among islands that open secretly onto other seas, into other worlds which I entered, following it. The language of charts is the visible in outline, the beach or cape or spit of land, the cliff face conspicuous from a coasting ship, the reef just breaking, the bright littoral that encloses every island translated to a black line by the flowing pen, the white foaming rock to a blackened star. This is their language, but it is not their subject: charts chart the numinous and are the textbooks for a certain kind of yearning.

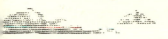

But let us turn back to the Santa Maria's low gallery where Columbus sits in the shadow of the deck
and awaits our full attention, a soft tipped brush
poised above the island of arrival. Behind the black
apostrophe that marks the crescent of the beach,
the bay the ships are sailing into, he lays down a
preliminary wash of island green, vivid and translucent. And now, to show this first anchorage and its
depth, uncoils with his pen a length of the lead and
line. It is the small inshore lead, armed with tallow,
so scrupulous in detail you can see the strips of
leather at the two and three fathom marks, the
white rag at five, the red at seven.

It is not disappointment, but surprise to find so
little of what he had been thinking of, ghosting in
on the making tide to a broad and shining bay. The
bosun sounds the still water. At every fall the lead
marks its own centre; ripples widening outward
link with those before and after, the ship's course
marked by this light chain. His singing chant comes
back to them from the woods behind the beach,
strong and clear and startling after a month on the
echoless ocean. And with the echo come all the
other sounds, a flood of the particular; instead of
the dull percussion of the waves, they hear their
own breath as it escapes them, and as it is drawn in,

with it comes the dizzy scent of pine, overwhelm-
ing, lucid; the rustling of the palms that line the
beach and just now begin to shift and sway in the
first trace of the morning breeze breaks in upon
them as though upon their sleep, sibilant and dis-
tinct; a brook that clatters across the beach on the
far shore rings like a bell; across the hollow bay, the
green of the forest keens, birdsong; the sea-worn
sails furl like sheering silk; each thing astonishing
in its clarity and separateness glistens under the
light of the senses returning, it seems, one by one,
the knot of the voyage that bound them up suddenly loosened. The morning is still, the bay to all
appearances deserted: no town, no village, not
even a clearing or a path presents itself. True,
mixed in with the scent of the forest warming in
the morning sun, there might be the sour trace of
an extinguished fire, and there is at least the possibility of fishing nets draped like shadows to dry
among the shadows higher up the beach.

This is nothing that he had expected.

But consider, reader, in this brief hiatus (for the
bay is not deserted, nor is it still for long: if you look
here, off the island's southern point, you will see
where Columbus has already painted, in a dense
wash of blue bice, the shadow of the morning
breeze that picks up the islands one by one all along

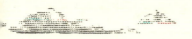

this archipelago, bright shells gathered in a palm of
wind), consider how this prospect – the running
brook of sweet water, the solace of the scented air,
the flowers and the earth, the white strand and safe
harbour – how this prospect might allay any disappointment over unmet expectations, and instil instead a sense of wonder in one so long at sea and so
far from home. The place might seem magical.

And indeed, when the first trace of morning
breeze turns the mirror of the bay to the wall and
the ships swing to and set their anchors, several
young men and a girl emerge from the porous wall
of trees and slough off the leaves' green shade,
stepping naked into the sunlight. Their movements
are easy and unhurried and clothed in light. They
slide a boat out from a shaded lee and into the water to the depth of their thighs where they slip into
the narrow hull to take up their flashing oars. The
winged hull moves just a breath above the surface
of the bay where it leaves no wake, despite its swift-
ness, and the paddles feather nothing but the
bright air. The paddlers are decorated with
cochineal, yelloe, black, their skin, myrrh slightly
darkened. Behind them, the island itself is extrava-
gant, a green gem set in gold, banded by a line of
white and then by turquoise (fine ground azurite),
and set in a deep blue wash of ocean. When they

come up to the ships and speak, their voices are like the senseless soft chattering of birds.

But despite the chart's excesses (gold dissolved in ox-bile brightens some sections of the beach, and lapis lazuli deepens the inland lakes), the ships do not stay for long at this first island. When Columbus rows ashore and, unsteady after a month on the pitching sea, climbs carefully backwards over the bluff bow of the ship's boat onto the sand, he looks down to see the toe of his narrow shoe pointing seaward (and still westward); this we may, as he does, interpret as a sign, his footprint clear in its declaration of departure not arrival. Today and tomorrow they do take time to enjoy the beach and eat a local meal of conch fritters and iguana tail, cassava bread, and carry out a little trade in beads (for braiding in the hair), and in the colour red. And Columbus makes a formal proclamation which, in a word, lays claim to this one island. But the ceremony of arrival is muted, a small speech in a large hall, and all parties seem unsure of the dimensions of their gestures, whether of conquest or of greeting: the one invents a ritual for surprise, the other for arrival at a place they cannot recognize.

Columbus is working by dead reckoning, and dead reckoning finds its meaning in motion only; a careful balance between expectation and observa-

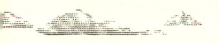

tion, it defines where the ship is, always and only in terms of where it has been and is going. Consider the instruments he has at his disposal: the compass in its binnacle, that precipitous enclosure; the ampoletta, or sand glass, that lays down its golden path through time; the knotted log-line that measures out the ship's speed through the water; and the lead and line that leads them through the brailled shallows. He is not equipped for standing still. And so it should be no surprise that we find him even now, on this evening of the first day, mixing burnt umber with egg-white (beaten and settled) for the hulls, myrrh lightened with yelloe for the sails lit by the morning sun, and white lead for the water cresting at the bows. Look. He has already set the three ships into another day and westward under full sail, their shadows billowing before them. Vermilion pennants unfurl at the mastheads.

It is just dawn and the bows bear down on the still midnight west. Behind them the first island has flattened to a silhouette against the eastern sky when the sun lifts free and burnishes the empty sea before them. The guides he has taken lean against the gunwale and sweep the horizon from the south to the northwest, calling out between them a litany of one hundred islands that lie just beyond their sight; the ships sail out among them.

By noon they arrive at the first, the ragged hem of a flag left flying for a season. The lookout spends all afternoon at the masthead describing the script of its reefs, which Columbus carefully transcribes along with the softer brushstrokes of the sandbars and the shifting colours of the currents themselves where the colder water rises out of the well of the ocean onto the shallow banks and opens like an eye around the torn island. Tonight the three ships lie at anchor under its western cape. The sun goes down and sets the night sky into motion high above them. Beneath, there is only the one fire, glittering on the beach. Reader, the day itself has been an island. Columbus has not fixed this place among the stars, nor this moment in their wheeling. Below in his trunk, the quadrant, cut from ebony, an ivory scale and brass plumb, rests on its side in the starless velvet night of its fitted case, its silken thread coiled round it. Tonight, the constellation of islands he has so far charted, each with its beach, each with its fire, will slip out beneath the dark hulls of their sleep and adrift on the black current, out onto the night sea. In the morning they will wake to the same sweet wind that blows tonight and frays the edges of their dreams, and before they set off again, Columbus will draw the three ships,

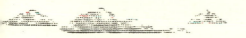

though at anchor, with their sails set and the waters coursing by them.

The chart, despite careful observations and clear record, despite the endless calculations, the rigour of the triangle, the accounting for current, for course, for course made true, despite the shrewd approximations of speed and speed over the ground, and constant soundings, can fix his land-falls only locally, and only in relation to one an-other, not to the world at large, or, for example, to a home on another sea that lies somewhere far to the east and beyond the long passage. Its method must flatten the earth's sphere, and so unstrings and straightens the imagined longitudes. No, al-though the chart is oriented to the world and to its north, it is not in the world, it is a world apart.

And perhaps to this we can credit the discomfort of the solitary canoeist they plucked from the sea an hour ago and brought, canoe and all, within the belly of the ship. He greets their mimed questions concerning gold mines and oriental dress with plain astonishment, and is not pleased to recognize his own island caught in the chart's coarse seine. He is polite, but suspicious of the proferred bread and sweet molasses, and it is with great relief that he sees this next island, which he was headed for,

lift long and low and familiar just on the edge of
the approaching dusk.

The ships arrive too late to anchor, the shallows
already shuttered against the falling night, and so
are standing off until dawn. Columbus watches
from the rail as the canoeist leaves them, skirts the
harbour's point and beach, and paddles into the
deeper darkness the veiled island has put on. All
night, his eyes inflamed with lack of sleep and looking, he traces absently the invisible currents that
brush along the shore and touch the sails and fill
them.

In the morning they turn south and then, all day,
sail eastward, and to these next islands, like the fragments of a broken vessel from which the evening
breeze spills out. Here the dew is scented as it falls,
and all night the scent of many flowers they do not
know the names for is tangled in the air.

They sail on and keep, as it were, first one hand
and then the other trailing along the leafy wall, the
beach where they do not land or cross. There are
many islands and many ways among them, and by
now they are lost in repetition, each one different,
each the same. (And lost to us too, reader, the first
already closed in upon itself, its few artifacts, shards
of clay or steel, the broken bowl, the hatchet with

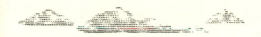

the broken blade, lapped in folds of sand.) By day
the lookouts harvest them from azure limbs, one by
one, like ripened fruit. It is the season of the falling
stars, and tonight the sailors watch them coming
down all around from the tree of darkness. In the
twining voyages of their sleep, they swear that there
are voices, perhaps the pink throated shells singing
on the tide, perhaps the scattered islands that they
lie anchored by drumming in the night wind, or the
shifting of their golden sands. They carry on, turning and turning in a sea starred with rocks and cays
without number, sailing now, even at night, led not
by what they find but by what eludes them. All this
goes into the chart.

From here the line of the journey turns south.
Across a shallow bank and a broad straight, the
brass dividers flash along the course line and prick
the chart where flying fish scissor by the hulls, their
backs and ribbed wings pearled in the domes of the
stern lanterns' light and in tonight's light rain. The
ships cross over.

When dawn fills in this next harbour, a party
goes ashore. Say that we go with them; three or
four together, we leave the jostling ship for an hour
and climb up to a village concealed by a scrim of
trees. Its inhabitants have all fled – the birds, for a

moment startled into silence, mark their going just
as we walk into the clearing. You step alone into the
doorway of the first house and into its airy darkness. It is cool and pleasant under the thatched
roof of palm fronds, and as your eyes adjust you see
that the interior is well ordered, like a ship: hooks
and nets and gear are coiled along the walls, the
floor is carefully swept and clear except for a
hearth of flat stones at the centre where a cooking
fire still smoulders; beside it a calabash of water
glints in the light that pours in from an opposite
doorway. Around you the fine nets of hammocks
slung to posts emerge from the shadows. Then you
notice the smooth bright pieces of shell that hang
by threads from the roof pole and rafters and, dis-
turbed by the recent commotion of departure, turn
slowly just above your head. You are just reaching
up to still them when something shifts behind you,
by the door, and you wheel to see a dog beside the
threshold – you must have brushed by it when you
entered, startled by the darkness, and now you remember the touch of fur against your leg. It eyes
you warily but does not bark or rise. You touch
nothing and go on your way.

From the water, the village again disappears.
They sail out close by it and set their course down
along the long steep coast. "My tongue could not

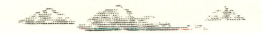

tell nor my pen describe," exclaims Columbus. He
has no adjectives left, and as if in compensation he
begins to clutter the shore with names for every
headland, bay, and river, every harbour, point, or
cove. He writes them out from the shore in his flowing script wherever the ships pass, and the waters
darken behind them as they go as if from the long
dark fingered gusts that press down from the high-
lands. As he writes, increasingly he senses within his
hand and pen an imminence that stirs as though
within a chrysalis, the urgent 'X' that will end this
outward voyage and anchor these wheeling islands
to a world he knows. But first the ships press on
across another strait, this one silvered by winds that
back and veer. The ship's boy sounds it with a skip-
ping stone that glints across the glittering surface
before it disappears; down and down it sinks, first
forgetting colour, then forgetting light. Beneath
them, the ocean floor has divided and dropped
away to nothing before it rises steeply on the other
side to meet their fumbling anchors in the waters
of Hispaniola.

If the chart has, by now, become like a garden
enclosed, Columbus draws this next island as its
pure lily and perfect rose. Here he sketches in familiar woodlands of oak and pine and arbutus to
cloak the island's sloping shoulders to the shore;

villages and ordered towns; hills like those of Tenerife, but higher; cool and deep ravines that open into secret plains of cultivated wheat and barley like the plains of rich Cordoba. The sea is full of salmon. And along this shore, for the first time, he draws people crowded at the water's edge holding up their gifts and articles of trade. Now the ships are ballasted at every harbour that they pass with parrots, cotton, water, bread and yams.

And today in the bay he calls St. Tomas, Columbus will receive an ancient mask of polished wood mounted on a cotton belt of intricate design. This mask has been on a journey too. For two hundred years it has winged its way through the islands, east and north, sometimes by canoe, sometimes worn by a man walking overland, sometimes slung from a ridge pole near a fire's light. Salt spray has cleansed it, the dew and falling rain have smoothed it, evening has closed its eyes and morning opened them, always on a new island. Today it is on the move again, laid in a basket of scented grass in the stern of a great canoe. The coast hurtles by, bay, cove, island, mangrove, the fifty paddlers silent at their work. River mouths open and speak to it in passing: "Oh, you who we carried in our arms"; rocks and sharp shells sing out to it from the crashing shale: "Child, it was we who shaped you"; the

forests whisper, all afternoon the canoe flies by
them and the wind through the leaves whispers:
"Brother, Brother, hear us." The salt waves hiss.
The canoe carries on.

If you, reader, perhaps with these same entreat-
ies echoing in your ears, stooped now to take this
ancient artifact from its basket, you would be su-
prised by its weight and texture. It is carved of
lignum vitae, and it is the size and heft of a human
heart, the surprising weight of stone or water. Turning it over in your hands you would feel the gloss of
its sweet oil, brought out by the afternoon sun, and
would also remark that recently (only yesterday in
fact were the gold rings beaten into foil) cataracts
of gold had formed across its eyes; its ears, nose,
tongue and eyes all gilded over the beautiful dark
wood.

It is evening when the emissary finally arrives, his
paddlers sagging on their benches, a torch burning
at the bow. He speaks a golden thread of words
across the dark water from his canoe and then
comes up to the ship to make his presentation. Columbus takes up the mask and belt, he holds it up –
with its flashing eyes, its winged brow, its stopped
ears and tongue, it could seem an ominous gift, but
Columbus's heart is light. He straps it on, the ancient mask, and sets aside all doubt that the next

bay, around the next headland, is the bay of prom-
ises. The ships set blindly out.

In the drama of discovery, the shape of its first act is
always comic: whatever you do, it is the right thing
to do. You are always moving forward. Consider, for
example, the wavering course of the Santa Maria as
it makes its way in close under the hills of Hispaniola just past midnight this Christmas morning. It is
calm, and the ship ghosts in closer and closer on
the whispering tide. What wakes them from their
sleep is not motion, but its absence.

There are two kinds of groundings. One is a sudden exclamation of rock or mud or coral against
the hull. The masts will whip forward with surprising suppleness, blocks, deadeyes, parted rigging
will singe the air, and on the recoil the decks may
buckle and the bulkheads shiver like glass. If the
bank is steep, the ship will sink in moments, with all
hands lost; or, it may fix itself on a spur of rock or a
sloped shelf while some of the crew, crazed by the
sudden pounding of the waves – the sea turned
suddenly against them – fling themselves into the
surf that opens around them. In this kind of
grounding your response is instantaneous and savage. You find yourself scrabbling to save the ship as
though it were your own body; you work without

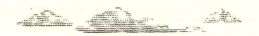

thought, often with exceptional strength, and without pain or even an awareness of, for example, the coldness of the water, cuts or splinters in your hands and feet, or the bruises that spread like tidal pools under the skin of your ribs or shoulders.

In the second kind, even the realization that you are aground may come slowly, your understanding taking shape as you sense a coldness creep into the hull beneath your feet, and as you look for and recognize the other signs: the regular slow slatting of a halyard, silenced; the deadened response of the rudder; the card of the compass fixed; and finally, a new heaviness in your step as you move across to the rail to look down and be sure.

The wreck of the Santa Maria is of this second kind. The ship's boy is alone at the tiller and his eyes are narrow and near sleep, lulled by the light hull's gentle rocking. When the stem touches gently on the bank, the sound it makes is so slight, just the other side of waking, so light he thinks it could be footfalls forward, or a coil of rope dropping from its pin. Then the sound again. And this time they have lifted up the bank and stuck fast, and the hull has turned to stone. The tide is on the ebb, and really, even now, the crew still sleeping, the boy still standing at the helm as though still sailing on, the stars still in their ordinary places, it is too late.

In either kind of grounding there is a threshold that you cross without knowing it. In the first you do not recognize it because the cresting wave of blood pumped to your head, your straining arms and hands prevents you, and in the second it is often crossed before you can shake off the sense of disbelief, like heavy sleep, and properly assess your situation. While you work to float the ship, sending out the kedging anchors warped to the mastheads, casting off the water barrels stored on deck, rolling the heavy guns and shot over the side, the spare anchors, the spare spars, the spars themselves, and finally cutting free the heavy masts, at some point you discover that you have been working all along in conjunction with the rocks and waves that press and grind the hull below the waterline, helping to dismantle the very ship it was your intention to save. Then all hope ebbs from you, and with it all your strength. At this point often comes a sense of calm, and if the sea is still, as it is tonight, you may notice for the first time the chuckling of the waves as they move further and further down the hull on the ebbing tide. And that the wind is picking up.

When Columbus has time again to settle by his chart, he will not represent the wreck caught in its bright aureole of foam, but instead the fort they are building even now on shore out of its salvaged tim-

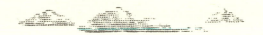

bers. Listen to the heavy ropes running again through the blocks, the spars raised into scaffolding; listen to the hammer blows that follow the beating of the drum; listen to the singing anvil and the roaring forge that shape nails, hooks and hinges, bars and bolts out of the ship's chainplates, gudgeons, pintals, out of its ironwork and bronze; listen to the axes swinging at the mazy roots of the mangrove, clearing a perimeter; and the pickets driven into the soft earth and bound; the barrels rumble on the ramps; the livestock shriek in their new pens; listen to the shouts of the men working in the morning and on into evening too; they lean into the cables and heave, dragging all of this across the beach.

It is perhaps inevitable that the fort resemble a little the ship from which it is built. The carpenters are first shipwrights, and their stock retains its shape, though pressed to another service. Columbus, seated comfortably on the beach the day before departure, draws it with its prow turned westward across the cresting waves of the island's green interior. The wreck was providential, and on the chart it flies the brightly coloured flags of promised commerce and of colonial Spain.

At dawn the two ships lie stern to stern, one the shadow of the other, one ashore and pointing west,

one bringing in its anchors and headed east to-
wards home. Columbus, his table set up now on-
board the crowded Nina, turns with the rest to look
back and sees the crew he has left ashore gather on
their parapet and wave fair passage; their raised
hands flicker in the early light as the sun climbs
over the eastern rail and stains them and then the
sails. On the Nina they feel the deck lift beneath
their feet with the first long wave from Africa that
lifts the bows then blooms along the beach behind.
Braced against it, Columbus leans once more to the
chart and marks this harbour with a cross, and beside it "Navidad." The ship's boy turns the glass and
sings.

TRANSLATION:

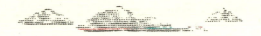

*He departed three hours before daybreak*
*from the gulf that he called the Golfo de*
*las Flechas with wind from the land, and*
*later with a west wind, taking the ships ...*
*northeast by east, toward Spain.*

## THE RETURN

This voyage is made under the sign of Roman Janus,
two-faced god of beginnings, quadropticon,
tollkeeper of the tongued gate on this half-built
bridge between worlds, circumspect patron of the
drafty doorway in which these sailors hesitate, Janus
of the threshold who is always coming and going,
prince of paradoxes, the proprietor of pauses, god
of the in-between, singularly sighted Janus, who
looks both ways at once: forward and backward,
past and future, east and west, recto and verso – all
simple in his double sight. And looking thus, what
does Janus see? The scope of his authority is as wide
as the sea itself, which, likewise, is a domain between domains. And it is from this watery vantage
that he charts the numberless departures and arriv-
als that clamour at its shores. He sees that the sea is
pure verb, and yet our voyages across it take on a

certain shape, a certain pattern which is the pattern of our thought and speech. They are voyages of discovery, and discovery predicates.

Today, just past the ides of his own month, Janus is filled with futurity, and so takes special note of the two leaky caravels coming into sight at dawn before his western eyes. Wave tossed and lightly ballasted with souvenirs, the two ships make their way eastward and toward home where already it is afternoon. And, at that face, Janus sees that all the harbours of Europe (though they do not know it yet) are waiting for the incredible news the two ships bring across the murmuring sea. On every pier in every port sit the sentinels, the old men, waiting. They wait through the lazy hours of the afternoon and through the end of the day, waiting and watching the lowering sun at the horizon's lip even after the return of the fishermen, their sons, and at nightfall they wait and listen to the breakwater stones lisp against the tide.

The two ships are bringing tokens with them. Shut up under the tongues of their hatches, parrots, insane and beautiful in their captivity, repeat an endless litany of invective against the darkness; strange masks made of gold stare fixedly in safe chests, emptying their eyes into a darkness crowded

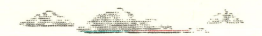

by iconic shadows – thrown together by the slanting ship, they have lost all propriety; other boxes are filled with bows, wood-tipped arrows and some tipped with bone or teeth, spear shafts, stone zemies, manioc scrapers and presses, bowls of wood, balls of rubber, spools of cotton, calabashes, sea shells; deep in the hold, plants with mistaken identities grow moldy in protest – medicinal Chinese rhubarb that is not, aloe that is not, cinnamon that is not – also the docile and resistant tubers which, being unknown, carry with them only their own expectations, the potato, the aje or yucca root, among them the fierce peppers that shrivel and dry but keep their secret, and there is maize, yellow and black and red; and deeper still, lumps of black ore flecked with fool's gold chuckle at the old joke. And there are the captives without number, bound by the senseless and the unfamiliar.

These are only the most evident of the tokens the ships are bringing with them. There are others cocooned in the folds of stored sails, and the sailors themselves carry still others, stealthy, winding through their blood and nerves, and still others, the silent spirilla of stories of unaccountable wealth and cruelty and happiness, of the simple life, and of aunciente libertie, branch across their palms and wait to be told. The ships are full, are riddled by the new and strange. And yet, except for the muffled incantation of the parrots, they have fallen into silence; indeed, the sea itself is still. The captives in the hold cannot speak of where they are, and if they could we could not hear them, and the sailors cannot speak of what they've seen. They have brought with them the first entries in a new lexicon:

> *aje, aji, anona,*
> *batata,*
> *cacique, canoa, caona, casavi,*
> *guacamayo, guanin,*
> *hamaca,*
> *maiz,*
> *nitaino, nozay,*
> *tuob*

– they have brought with them the first entries in a new lexicon, but they have not learned its grammar; the new words lie on their tongues, inert as stones, and silence them.

And so this episode is marked only with the muttering of the waves. This evening the old men have gone home disgusted from the pier heads to tell tales of their youth enlivened by exotic places they have not seen but dreamed of, and the sailors on

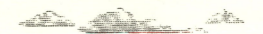

the two ships imagine their dry old age and try to think of where they've been. This pleases diabolic Janus by its unity, and the good god of beginnings, seeing nothing new, shuts all his eyes and, the door left ajar for the west wind, stretches out across his ocean threshold and sleeps.

## THE THRESHOLD

And it is the west wind that wakes him.

It begins like a promise couched in a listening ear. Then on the first day the sky lowers to a narrow margin and the waves build and become terrible. On the second day the seams open, and the ships forsake their easting along with all hope. On the third day they sight land but cannot reach it. On the fourth day they reach land, but their anchors do not hold, and they are blown back to sea. The ships fall and fall from the sheer waves through a whirlwind of driving rain and spray where the elements themselves become uncertain: fire, water, salt, or air. Shaken from their senses, the sailors litter the securest corners of the deck and lash themselves down in all the attitudes of the dispossessed; lashed behind the bulwarks, they turn inward and meditate on fixed particulars: a bubble of tar that has worked out of a deck seam, a stream of water that frays and tears from a singing sheet or stay, the shifting note of the wind itself. The ships' boats have been smashed and scattered, broken rigging flies in ragged pennants from the masts and yards, the decks are awash, the ships near foundering.

And below in his cabin, Columbus is writing a letter. With him are the cooper and the cabin boy. They make a strange tableau for the final curtain. The lamp has already gone out once and been relit. It is swinging wildly. Columbus is half standing at his table, one foot braced against a trunk. The cooper, his back against the bulkhead, has secured the first hoops for a small barrel and now prepares the lid, and the cabin boy is melting wax. Columbus is writing a letter to be posted at death's door. Into the letter he disburdens the little bark of his mind of its cargo of names: San Salvador, Santa Maria de Concepcion, Fernandina, Isabella, Babeque, Cabo Hermosa, Las Islas de Arena, Río de la Luna, Río de Mares, Río del Sol, Cabo de la Laguna, Cabo de Torres, Cabo Alto y Bajo, Cabo Alpha y Omega, Río del Oro, Valle del Paraíso – names that could be the names of anywhere – San Salvador, in remembrance of the Divine Majesty, extensive Juana with its huge harbour, Española, lovely and rich for planting and sowing, for breeding cattle, for building towns … These he inscribes carefully on parch-

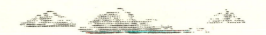

ment, sets and seals them in a cake of wax, shuts
them up tightly in a barrel, and casts them adrift on
the wind-lashed and endless sea.

Perhaps you, reader, feel that this resort to messages in bottles is a vain, a hopeless gesture. But
look back just now through Janus' darkened doorway and you can see there before his western eyes
that it is mid-morning and that, in his canoe, a solitary fisherman is sleeping, rocked gently by the
quickening waves and the morning breeze that
skirts the green hills and throws them into relief,
and by the long pull of the ground swell rising over
the bank edge of blue water. This fisherman is
dreaming that a small round fish has come and
swallowed all the islands, even the big ones.

And so what of this barrel of names that it can
swim into the sleep of such a distant dreamer? Even
as we speak it sets off eastward and out of sight of
the torn ships, making its way through the steep
and cresting seas toward Spain as sure and buoyant
as a tiny leviathan. And of what significance is its
cargo, addressed to the Spanish sovereigns? At the
moment when Columbus casts it out onto the troubled sea, he is rightly fearful for his own safety and
the safety of his ships. He means to save the idea of
his discovery, attested by the letter sealed in the
cake of wax, even if the discoverer himself is lost,

and it buoys his spirits to think of the little barrel making its way shoreward to be cast up on the beach and found by a man drying his nets or, better, hauled from the sea like a golden fish of promise. In the end, it is not the ships or their admiral but the barrel itself that is lost forever. Waterlogged within the hour, it sinks out of the wind's way into the endless silence that waits just below the sea's surface. Here it circles gently in the vast encircling currents, to the east, south, west, north, and back again to the east and south months later or even years, repeating itself again and again in the Atlantic round, its writing pristine and hermetic in its waxen seal.

But we can chart the letter's course another way. Its other journey is the journey of an idea outward into language. "There I found very many islands: San Salvador, Santa Maria de Concepcion, Fernandina, Isabella, Juana ...": Columbus inscribes his string of names across the parchment.

Is it this inscription that troubles the canoeist in his troubled dream: the flowing script, serpentine, transformative, its influence reaching so far westward that it disturbs the little vessel of his sleep? A sinuous cold frond of current brushes against the bottom of his canoe and wakes him. When he

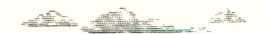

wakes, he finds the islands still spread out before him, white-brimmed, wind-shadowed, blue-hilled and familiar, but he does not feel the sudden relief of waking from a dream to find the world set aright, but utter sadness.

But there is yet another course that the letter takes, and this time it is on a journey inward. The storm has not abated, but has driven Columbus' ship north to the shores of Portugal. Just after nightfall, the lookout, the one man spared from work at the pumps, sights by a break in the clouds and the full moon the Rock of Sintra and, beyond it, the smooth-flowing waters of the Tagus, entry-way to Lisbon. All of the sails but one have been blown out, and the wind drives them down all night on the lee and broken shore; all night they make to windward, losing ground, but slowly. With first light they ease out of the wind's eye, scudding wildly for the channel's narrow gap, one yard slung low, and the one sail so bellied with the driving wind and spray it turns translucent as the river wa-ter whose fraught traces now touch the keel and whose sweetness the sailors taste in the spume-crazed air. And then they are over the bar and through the breach.

And nothing happens.

By nine o'clock they are at anchor in the river below Lisbon. The day is clear but windy. A hawk hangs in the air above the river valley. On the bank some belled goats forage by a white cottage, tended by a girl in green. Two fishermen row out to speak with them.

But there is the letter. Its ragged corner is just visible at the throat of Columbus' doublet. He finished writing it this morning to the incredible sound of goat's bells and to fragments of a girl's singing carried across the water on the wind. (It is the same letter, apart from this morning's addendum, that is, at this very moment drifting westward in its barrel, caught in the outflowing current of this same river.) Columbus is reaching for it now. We see that it is sealed and addressed. He hands it to a messenger who already holds a small leather purse of coins. The messenger is listening to the instructions the Admiral is giving him. He is putting on his broad-brimmed hat. He is mounting his horse; his flashy boots slide into the stirrups. He is setting off along the road to the interior and to the Spanish Court at Barcelona on the shores of the inland sea.

But messenger, wait, have you no curiosity? Messenger, before you are out of sight around this

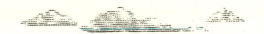

bend in the road and over the brow of the hill, why
not let your horse rest awhile and nibble at the
river grasses and shoots of the ferns here on the
Tagus' lush banks? You have a long journey
through the high and rocky barrens before you,
and all around you now the irises are blooming. Do
you hear the doves cooing in the glade? Stop here a
moment. Refresh yourself. Unseal the letter and
be, yourself, the first to discover what is in it.

And so he does. Under Janus' divided gaze he
sits down beside a narrow bridge in the shade of a
laurel tree and takes the letter from his pouch. It is
light, one sheet folded twice, and he sees that the
seal is thick and poorly fixed, and easily undone.
He moistens the parchment with his breath and
warms the waxen seal between his palms until it lifts
unbroken from the flap. And then, the afternoon
sun slanting through the laurel's branches and dap-
pling in a lozenged shade the page in his hands, he
reads ...

THE LETTER

and reading thus, is transported to a garden.

Where he sits the bridge before him had been
barren stone, but now it is bordered by blue hem-

lock and pillared with cone-shaped cypress trees, while along its balustrade creeps the tendrilled vine, pliant-footed ivy twined. A company of willows haunts the river bank with shadows, and further on the summer foliage of the oak, the beech and soft linden surrounds a pleasant glade. In thirty-three measured steps the messenger ascends to the crest of the hump-backed bridge from where his gaze contracts the whole prospect of the garden laid out before him, its vast perimeter marked in by mountains of a thousand shapes. Before him an avenue of palms of six or eight varieties leads from the bridge's foot to the garden's centre where it meets a second thoroughfare that cuts the garden through and makes of it three regions; each region is mazed with hedges (not ordered but ordered by the eye to seem in their lax symmetry as dense and fine and perfect as Indian carpets, but woven of scented cedar, box, clipped bay and myrtle), these opening onto groves of great pines and varied orchards, each orchard marvellous in extent and fruitfulness and fed by clattering brooks that stem from a single fountain near the garden's centre, scented by rough mastic, lit by the lily and the rose.

The messenger crosses over to the bridge's other side. When he steps into the garden, he is embraced by the most temperate of breezes which

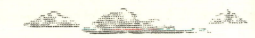

leads him from the avenue of stately palms to wan-
der among trees very green and more beautiful
than any he has ever seen. Solicitous fruit trees,
some bearing two or three varieties together, bend
into his hands their ripened fruit while blossomed
still. At every glade and mounded garden that he
passes, the gentle people of the place rouse themselves from sleeping or from their pleasant work
and, making mute signs of homage, bring him
gifts of what they have of water, cotton, gold, a
kind of bread, the produce from their common
plots, stalks of rare rhubarb, chips of cinnamon
and aromatic cedar, of which value they seem in-
nocent, accepting nothing in return. The messenger hears within a stand of taller trees the forest-
muted song of the nightingale, an indigo thread
drawn through the wood's green shade and
through the song and chatter of a thousand other
birds. This he follows. Deep in under the shadow
of the green canopy, feathers flash through the
veil of trees in primary reds and greens and blues.
A snapped twig sends above his head a startled
flock of pigeons that breaks like thrown water
against the leafy roof and sky and leaves the enclosure, for an instant, silent. The messenger calls
out and is answered by a hundred echoing voices.
Then, deep within a darkened copse, the nightin-

gale begins again, and he thinks he should stay there forever within the circle of the sound within the shadow of the wood.

Here the messenger lets the letter fall against his knee. Each thing in the garden is a marvel to him, and yet the garden's form is familiar, its intersecting avenues, its vast perimeter marked in by a deeper wilderness where burn signal fires and, beyond, the drumming of the mountains. The garden is familiar to him and yet strange – but it is not the strangeness of the new he feels, but of a new domain of déjà vu. Everything is as expected, and yet remote. He cannot taste the black cherries that he crushes on his tongue, and the varied blossoms, though sweet, carry only a general, a universal scent. The water in the brooks is cold and fresh, but so distilled it has no savour, and the apple has no heft.

Here the messenger lets the letter fall against his knee. Behind the letter fall the shadows. Evening floods the river's upper reaches and floods and fills the valley. He breaks off a laurel wand above his head and stands and stretches. For a moment he looks westward, then mounts his horse and leaves behind the ocean's roar at the river's mouth. This is the end of the beginning, and Janus, heaving a diaphonic sigh, also turns away and faces for a while to the North and to the South.

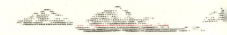

This letter is not the first that the messenger has previewed, thereby to judge in advance his welcome (to choose carefully the time of his arrival, whether to make his presentation in public, private, or the company of friends), and so it is not with a credulous but a critical eye that he has set about the task of reading. He understands at once that this is no garden but the Garden of Eloquence he has been wandering in, itself an allegory for his own desire. The letter is lettered with the alphabet of ownership, and it is by this lettering that the strangeness of the garden is made familiar, that the foreign is brought home, by this that all its varied pleasures are figured within the frame of his own yearning. In the alphabet of ownership *A* stands for *aleph*, which is a word for ox, or for the yoke, the furrow and the plough, for planting and sowing, for reaping, for husbandry, for fattening and slaughter; *B* is for *beth*, another word for house, for home, for all manner of edifices public and private, for hearthstone, well and wall; *gimel* is the word for *C*, and for camel, and means messages from abroad, commerce, empire. These are its A,B,Cs. The alphabet of ownership is the first lesson in the rhetoric of otherness, a messenger's stock in trade.

The second lesson is the parade.

Columbus is on the move as well. When the messenger stands and stretches, he is already three
days' sail up the coast from Lisbon and waiting for
the flood tide to carry him over the bar of Saltés.
When the messenger leads his horse across the narrow bridge, Columbus is furling his sails off Palos,
its houses guilded by the evening light, a crowd
gathering on the pier. And when the messenger
turns onto the good road at Talvera de la Reina,
Columbus is already on his way from Palos to
Seville. When the messenger rides down the hills
behind Barcelona and calls to the keeper of the
northern gate, Columbus, in Cordova, chafes
lightly between his forefinger and thumb the left
nipple of Beatriz Enríquez de Harana, she softly
moaning as he does, "my dove, my dove." When the
messenger rides through the gates of the city and
the palace gates, Columbus, breathless, takes her in
his arms and falls across the bed. And when the
messenger rides through the city gates and the palace gates and puts into the Queen's pale hands the
letter ... he sees it flower into a thousand copies of
itself and thread and twist into the bright banners,
the roped flowers, the ringing bells and snapping
flags of the Spring Parade. He sees the whole city

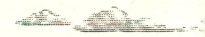

turned out to line the route, caught in the surge
and undertow of curiosity and dread; he sees the
limbs of the plane trees become leafy with children; he sees shutters thrown open, balconies over-
burdened, handkerchiefs waving, hats in the air,
dancing and singing, fancy ribbons and fancy dress;
and most clearly he sees himself. He sees himself
riding through the mazed streets to the city's gate
to take his place, the messenger, the first messenger, in the great parade. And when the messenger
sees all this, Columbus is already at the gate, and
the city's horsemen have ridden out to greet him,
the hooves of their eager horses clattering applause
all around him. Columbus is already at the gate,
and as he steps within the city's walls, his odd en-
tourage of souvenirs strung out behind him, the
welcoming cheer goes up all around him.

THE  SOUVENIRS

All through the streets you can hear Columbus
singing; he is singing to himself. Under his breath
he is singing, all the way to the Salo del Tinell,
where, under the span of its six broad arches, the
gathered court, the King and Queen, the Church-
men await his formal presentation. Light from the
courtyard slants in through a high window and illu-

minates them there, arranged in state at the centre of the dim stone hall, and Columbus himself now appears within its circle. Quoting from his own letter, he begins: "Although men have talked or have written of these lands, all was conjectural, without eye-witness, but amounted only to this, that those who heard for the most part listened and judged rather by hearsay than from even a small something tangible ...." And then, for testimony, he turns to the doorway, where, as he pronounces for each its native name, speculates on its character, use, and genus, the souvenirs are brought in: six Indians, nearly naked; a dozen parrots, some stuffed, some chained to perches; several trays of artifacts, fruits and samples; a small safe-chest of gold; a golden mask; a few pearls in a copper cup; some cotton cloth.

They are meant to stand for something else, the souvenirs, for something more, as islands in the sea suggest a foreign shore. But each, as it is brought in under the light, casts a shadow that, while it is the shadow of the thing itself, is the shadow of forgetting; each thing as it is named and brought forward opens a doorway into the empty room of loss. Watch Columbus as he turns, his hand held out toward the darkened door in the gesture that is a gesture both for beckoning and for letting go. Each

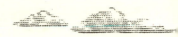

time he turns, he hears the name that he has spoken echo in the stone hall as though it were an image in a hall of mirrors. Each echo, as it stirs in the dimmer reaches of the room, announces, as it were, its own diminishment. The things themselves begin to waver in his sight and grow transparent; they seem to retreat beyond his reach. But all of this time, Columbus keeps singing, singing to himself until the stones themselves do seem to sing.

And this is where we leave him, where he stands under the ribbed roof of the Salo del Tinell. He is looking back, one hand held out behind him toward the stone doorway, his mouth just open, about to speak or perhaps speaking, but stopped here in time, and therefore silent – so silent that, if you listen, you can hear in the dim corners of the room, along the heavy wooden beams, the lintels, on the lips of the stone arches, deep in the recesses of the doors and their passageways, those shadows settling in, rustling in their nests, making room – yes, making room in a new world.

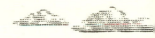

NOTES

PAGE 1: *Columbus primus inventor Indiae*, is plate vi of Theodor de Bry's *India Occidentalis*, vol. 4 (Impression Franco-furti, 1590). The engraving is reproduced here by courtesy of the Edward E. Ayer Collection, The Newberry Library, Chicago.

PAGE 3: Ovid sings of Orpheus the singer. (From *Metamorphosis*. Translated by Frank Justus Miller (London and New York: Loeb Classical Library, 1916), Vol. 2, p. 71.)

PAGE 8: According to Gordon Brotherstone, in his *Image of the New World* (Thames and Hudson, 1979), the Arawak tale describing the origin of Caribs was in turn adopted by the Caribs to explain the origin of Spaniards. In it, a girl contravenes a taboo by sitting on the ground while menstruating, and is impregnated by a snake, which her brothers then kill. After their birth, her snake children, who become Caribs (or Spaniards), ask for their father. She explains that her brothers have killed him and the hostilities commence.

PAGE 9: The questions for the interview of Alonso Sanchez are taken from entry 333 of Ludwig Wittgenstein's last book, *On Certainty*, on which he was working at the time of his death.

PAGES 13–15: Quotations here are taken from *The Travels of Sir John Mandeville* (N.Y.: Dover, 1964); Pierre d'Ailly's *Imago Mundi* (Boston, 1927); *Selections from the History of the World commonly called The Natural History of C. Plinius Secundus* (Essex: Centaur Press Ltd, 1962); and *The Travels of Marco Polo the Venetian* (London: J.M. Dent and Sons Ltd, 1926).

PAGE 22: This and other shipboard songs and prayers can be found in S.E. Morison, *Admiral of the Ocean Sea, a life of Christopher Columbus* (Boston: Little, Brown and Co, 1942) pp. 173 ff.

PAGE 27: This image is a detail of *Portuguese Carracks off a Rocky Coast*, attributed to Joachim Patnir (c. 1485), © National Maritime Museum, London.

PAGE 29: "Andando más, más se sabe" (the further one goes, the more one knows), writes Columbus, verifying by experience his early belief that the world is made up of six parts land and one part water. He is quoted here from *Select Documents Illustrating the Four Voyages of Columbus*, translated and edited by Cecil Jane. 2 vols. (London: Hakluyt Society, 1930) 2:43. See also Steven Greenblatt, *Marvelous Possessions*, (Chicago: University of Chicago Press, 1991) 88, for an interesting discussion of context.

PAGE 53: The Patonne is f. 51 in *Histoire Naturelle des Indies: The Drake Manuscript in the Pierpont Morgan Library*, translated by Ruth Kraemer, edited by Patrick O'Brien, Morgan Pierpont, Verlyn Klinkenborg (New York: W.W. Norton, 1996); The Pierpont Morgan Library, New York. MA 3900.

PAGE 75: The script shown here is copied from Columbus's original journal.

PAGE 94: The quotation is taken from the "Santagel Letter" written during a storm off the Azores on February 14 and 15th 1493 (*The Journal of Christopher Columbus*, translated by Cecil Jane, revised and annotated by L.A.Vigneras with an

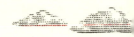

appendix by R.A. Skelton. [New York: Clarkson N. Potter, Inc., 1960]).

The Journal excerpts throughout are adapted largely from Dunn/Kelley *The Diario of Christopher Columbus's First Voyage to America, 1492–1493*, transcribed and translated by Oliver Dunn and James E. Kelley, Jr. [Norman: University of Oklahoma Press, 1989] with reference also to Jane (*The Journal of Christopher Columbus*, translated by Cecil Jane, revised and annotated by L.A.Vigneras with an appendix by R.A. Skelton [London: Anthony Blond and the Orion Press, 1960]) and, in the case of the note for October 11 and its signs of land, to Morison (*Journals and other documents on the life and voyages of Christopher Columbus*, translated and edited by S. Morison [N.Y.: Heritage Press, 1963]) for his branch of roseberries. (Both Jane and Kelley read the alternate "branch with barnacles" as more likely.) In selecting the excerpts, reference has also been made to Ferdinand Columbus' biography of his father (Colon, Fernando, *The Life of the Admiral Christopher Columbus by his son, Ferdinand*, translated and annotated by Benjamin Keen [New Brunswick, N.J.: Rutgers University Press, 1959]) and to the *Historia* of Bartolomé de las Casas (Bartolomé de las Cassas, *History of the Indies*, translated and edited by Andrée Collard [New York: Harper and Row, 1971]).

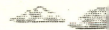

## ACKNOWLEDGMENTS

Much of my childhood was spent sailing up and down the coasts of Nova Scotia and Newfoundland with my family, often straining into the Atlantic fog for a bell or a light or a headland or the looming hull of a freighter, announced long since by the throbbing of its props, a sound just below hearing. From this perspective the world can seem at once uncertain and especially vivid and precious – a trace of sun-warmed spruce carried out on the raw air. It was a great place to begin thinking about the distances that inform this book. My thanks go to my mother, father, stepfather, and brother, who took me with them.

When a book as short as this takes as long to write as this one has, the list of people who have helped along the way can easily outweigh the text itself: gratitude has become, for me, a way of life during the writing of these pages. I would, however, like to acknowledge a few people especially: Kay Redhead, who thought it was a good idea; Ted Chamberlin, whose guidance in this project goes back to long before I understood it was a project at all; Martha Reynolds; Stan Fillmore; SaraJane, who made the first reading of the first page count; Steven and Gail Rubin for more than I can say; Lynda Rosborough for shelter; Linda, Meghan, Linnet, and Nigel; Derk Wynand and Marlene Cookshaw for their remarkable gifts as readers; Ricardo Sternberg; Michael Harris; Eric Ormsby; and Fiona. I would also like to acknowledge the journals in which parts of this text have previously appeared – *The Malahat Review*, *The Fiddlehead*, and *The Jean Rhys Review* – and, for the gift of time, Université Ste. Anne, the SSHRC, the Canada Council Explorations Program, and the Nova Scotia Arts Council. And I would like to thank Joan Harcourt, Joan McGilvray, and everyone at the McGill-Queen's Press for taking the book on and for doing it so beautifully.